Buddha's Guide to Fitness

The Path to Mindful and Holistic Health

Table of Contents

Chapter 1. Introduction

Delve into a transformative path to wellness like none other with our Special Report, "Buddha's Guide to Fitness: The Path to Mindful and Holistic Health". This enlightening journey integrates the profound wisdom of Buddhism with contemporary approaches to physical health, creating a unique mind-body fitness paradigm. This comprehensive guide unfurls not only the physical aspects of exercise, but also the mental and spiritual benefits to meditative movement, pushing the frontiers of conventional fitness wisdom. Radiating positivity and transcendental enlightenment, it might just be the catalyst you need to leap forward in your health journey. Don't miss this chance to sculpt the conscious health routine of your dreams - a wholesome blend of Buddha's teachings and modern fitness strategies are waiting for you in this uplifting special report. Tune into your spiritual self while enhancing physical stamina, flexibility, and strength. After all, your wellness journey is not just about changing the body, it's about awakening the soul!

Chapter 2. The Intersection of Fitness and Spirituality

The exploration of the intersection between fitness and spirituality is a unique journey. It involves not just looking at fitness as a routine set of exercises to keep the body healthy, but also understanding its implications on spiritual well-being. As Buddha once said, "To keep the body in good health is a duty, otherwise we shall not be able to keep our mind strong and clear." In seeking the harmony between body and mind, we come across a confluence of physicality and spirituality. This transformative path begins where the mundane exercises end, and the realm of spiritual awareness begins.

2.1. Embracing Holistic Wellness

Holistic wellness is a concept that sees the body, mind, and spirit as interconnected and interdependent entities. It goes beyond the mere physical fitness, touching the realms of mental and spiritual health in equal measures.

When we speak of holistic wellness, we don't look at the body as a separate entity from the mind and spirit. Instead, we see all three as interconnected pieces of a larger puzzle, all deeply affecting the other. We, therefore, aim to approach fitness with this integrated perspective in mind. Engaging in physical exercise or meditative practices alone will not provide the comprehensive benefits that a combined regimen of both can confer.

2.2. The Art of Meditative Movement

The concept of 'meditative movement' is an essential part of the disquisition. It involves integrating mindful awareness into physical movements. Such movements are undertaken with a deepened sense of self-awareness and a whole-hearted engagement, dissolving the mind-body boundary that is usually perceived in traditional fitness regimens.

For instance, forms of exercise like yoga and tai chi are often considered meditative movements. The focus is not merely on challenging the body but also on achieving mental clarity through the physical acts. The mindful engagement required during these practices instils a sense of calm, centeredness, and awareness that elevates the fitness routine from being a mere exercise to becoming a holistic wellness activity.

2.3. Understanding the Mind-Body Connection

The mind-body connection explains how our emotional, mental, social, and spiritual states can directly affect our physical health. More than just a philosophical idea, it is scientifically backed, with evidence showing that stress, depression, and other mental health conditions can lead to physical illnesses.

Fitness and spirituality intersect at this junction. Regular physical exercise can not only boost your physical health but also has been found to have a positive effect on mental health. On the other hand, spiritual practices like meditation can help in managing stress, thereby improving the quality of life. They bring about a calmness and clarity, helping us manage physical pain or illness more effectively, and thus solidifying the physical benefits of spiritual practices.

2.4. Fitness as a Spiritual Practice

One might wonder - how can fitness become a spiritual practice? It's not about following a religious doctrine or engaging in any form of ritualistic practice. Instead, it's about tapping into the greater power and potential within ourselves.

Each physical movement pushes our bodies to the brink, challenging our limitations. This act of constantly pushing and expanding our boundaries echoes the Buddhist principle of growth and progression. When pursued mindfully, with complete awareness and immersion into the act, the physical exercise transforms into a spiritual experience, enabling individuals to connect to their higher selves. Each stride, every lift, and all the stretches become a moving meditation, instilling a sense of inner balance and harmony.

2.5. Mindfulness and Exercise

Mindfulness is yet another intersection between fitness and spirituality. It's about fully engaging in the present moment, focusing on the movement of your body, paying attention to your breath, and recognizing each sensation as you exercise.

When we approach exercise in a mindful way, we shift our focus from merely achieving physical fitness to experiencing wholeness, from the rhythm of the breath to the strain of muscles, from the strength being forged to the silence that envelops the mind - every bit becomes a part of the fitness experience. Rather than seeing exercise as a laborious task, we start to see it as a profound expression of our existence.

2.6. A New Paradigm of Fitness

This intersection of fitness and spirituality shows us a new way of looking at health and well-being. It is a shift from the conventional approach, where the mind and body are seen as separate entities, to a holistic approach that acknowledges their interdependence.

To embody this new fitness paradigm is to nurture the body and the mind with equal emphasis, to acknowledge that mental and spiritual well-being is as important as physical health, and to recognize that these aspects are intricately connected.

So, as you embark on this holistic health journey, bear in mind that fitness is more than just physical workouts. It's a deeply spiritual practice that nourishes the mind, body, and spirit. And as you harness the power of this mind-body connection, you will step into a newer, more enlightened version of yourself. After all, as Buddha has wisely said, "Your body is precious. It is our vehicle for awakening. Treat it with care."

Chapter 3. Exploring Buddhism: Philosophy as a Fitness Guide

Buddhism's perspective on the human condition illuminates a path to holistic health that's rich, nuanced, and holistic. A fundamental understanding of this philosophy and its principles provides novel insights into how we can approach our physical and mental wellbeing. As we delve into this philosophy-driven fitness guidance, we should underscore the interconnectedness of body, mind, and soul - a concept intrinsically embedded in Buddhism.

3.1. Understanding the Four Noble Truths

The central tenets of Buddhism, the Four Noble Truths, provide the foundation for a comprehensive fitness and wellness approach. Summarizing, they suggest that: life is characterized by discomfort (Dukkha); discomfort arises from our desires and attachments (Samudaya); we can overcome discomfort by letting go of these attachments (Nirodha); and the path to doing so is through the Eightfold Path (Magga).

Comprehending the concept of Dukhka and translating it into our fitness journey translates to accepting that discomfort, in the form of strains or muscle aches, is an inherent part of the process. Understanding Samudaya pushes us to recognize unhealthy attachments to things like guilt-inducing strict diets, unrealistic body standards, or incessant comparisons. Nirodha teaches us to release these detrimental attachments for a more compassionate approach towards ourselves, thereby nurturing mental health. Finally, Magga prompts us to live holistically, observing right action, right mindfulness, and right effort, shaping our journey of fitness into one of personal growth and self-improvement.

3.2. Embracing the Eightfold Path

The Eightfold Path, as a segment of the Four Noble Truths, guides us towards moral, mindful and wise health choices. It encourages a balanced lifestyle, composed of right understanding, thought, speech, action, livelihood, effort, mindfulness, and concentration.

Right understanding and thought emphasize discernment over dietary choices and workout routines, rejecting quick-fix diets or strenuous exercise regimens that harm the body. Right speech, action, and livelihood push for honesty with oneself, preventing destructive behaviors such as overexercising or withholding food. Right effort, mindfulness, and concentration nurture the cognitive aspects of fitness, fostering consistent motivation, body-awareness, and focus during workouts.

3.3. Anicca: Embracing Impermanence

The Buddhist principle of Anicca, or impermanence, holds valuable insights for physical fitness. The human body is constantly changing. Muscles grow and recede; weight is gained and lost; injuries occur and heal. Accepting this volatility can cultivate resilience, transforming the way we perceive physical setbacks or slow progress in our fitness journeys.

3.4. Metta: Self-Love and Compassion

Metta, meaning loving kindness in Pali, is a cornerstone of Buddhist philosophy. Applying Metta to fitness demands compassion for oneself and one's body. It signifies letting go of body-shaming, embracing our physical selves with all the imperfections, and eschewing the societal pressure for a "perfect" body. It's about helping, not harming, our bodies through exercise and diet.

3.5. Mindfulness and Meditation

Mindfulness is the practice of being fully present in the moment, and meditation is a tool to cultivate mindfulness. Incorporating mindfulness boosts training efficiency by encouraging focus on form and breath, maximizing the benefits of each movement. Meditation aids in stress reduction and the enhancement of mental endurance, providing a balanced approach to fitness.

3.6. The Middle Way

The Middle Path teaches moderation in all aspects of life, including exercise and nutrition. This emphasizes adopting sustainable fitness patterns that evade extremes. It promotes intuitive eating, conscious consumption, regular movement, and adequate rest, forging a sustainable, positive relationship with fitness.

3.7. Ahimsa: Non-Violence and Peace

Buddha taught Ahimsa, or non-violence, which refers to peace towards all living beings, including oneself. From a fitness perspective, Ahimsa discourages vigorous routines that harm the body, pushing for workouts that strengthen without causing undue strain, and diets that nourish rather than deprive.

Exploring Buddhism as a fitness guide takes us on a reflective journey, revising our perspective on health. It prompts us to view fitness beyond physical parameters, incorporating mental growth, compassion, patience, and peace. Authentic health is an equilibrium of both physical agility and mental wellness, and this philosophy-infused approach gets us remarkably close to achieving that balance.

Chapter 4. Buddhist Approach to Physical Wellness

To truly comprehend the Buddhist approach to physical wellness, it is crucial to first establish an understanding of the fundamental principles of Buddhism that are directly related to health and wellbeing. Environmental harmony, balanced diets, mindfulness, and exercise are all elements of the Buddhist way of life that contribute to overall physical wellness. This chapter presents an exhaustive analysis of these principles, offering valuable insights for those seeking to incorporate this philosophy into their wellness journey.

4.1. The Middle Way

In Buddhism, the concept of the 'Middle Way' or 'Moderation' is a guiding principle. Gautama Buddha taught that moderation in all facets of life leads to a state of tranquility and balance, which in turn fosters physical wellness. This teaching can be applied to physical activity and diet among other areas.

It is important to understand that the Middle Way does not advocate for a lack of action or effort. Buddhists are encouraged to moderate their actions and thoughts, not eliminate them. Therefore, when considering physical wellness, individuals should aim for a state of balance - enough exercise to keep the body healthy and active, but not to the point of exhaustion or injury.

4.2. Mindfulness in Action

Buddha taught mindfulness as a method of dwelling in the present moment. This practice encourages individuals to experience and accept their physical sensations, emotions, and thoughts without judgment. Mindfulness brings heightened attention to the activity at hand, which provides a route to improved physical health.

Buddhist scriptures emphasize the importance of mindfulness during physical activity. This could be any activity—from gardening, walking to more formalized forms of exercise. The key is to be present in the moment, feeling every movement of the body and every breath taken, instead of focusing on future goals or past failures.

4.3. Mindful Eating

One of the most vital aspects of physical wellness in Buddhist philosophy is mindful eating. Buddhist teachings encourage a balanced diet, acknowledging that food is primarily meant for nourishing the body and supporting good health.

The practice of mindful eating involves paying keen attention to the food we consume, its flavors, its texture, its colors, and how our bodies react to it. It's about savoring each bite and expressing gratitude for the food. Also, this leads to the understanding of the role our dietary choices play in contributing to our physical health as well as environmental sustainability.

4.4. The Importance of Meditation

While meditation is often associated with mental and spiritual wellness, it is also a powerful tool for physical health. Firstly, regular meditation helps reduce stress and anxiety, which have a profound effect on the body's physical state. Meditating aids in lowering blood pressure, improving the immune system, and reducing chronic pain.

Moreover, certain forms of meditation incorporate physical movements, such as walking meditation or meditative yoga. These practices harmonize both the mind and body, creating a strong foundation for overall wellness.

4.5. The Principle of Non-Harm

The Buddhist principle of non-harm or 'Ahimsa' extends not only to others but also to oneself. This teaching encourages respect for the body and its needs, promoting actions that will keep it healthy and active. Regular exercise, adequate rest, and a balanced diet are all considered forms of self-respect, as they support the body's wellbeing.

In the Buddhist path to physical wellness, individuals learn to listen to their bodies and give them what they need. Exercise is not seen as a punishment, but rather as a way to honor the body.

In conclusion, the Buddhist approach to physical wellness lies in the intertwining of the mind and body. By embracing principles such as the Middle Way, mindfulness in action and eating, the importance of meditation, and the principle of non-harm, one can experience overall physical wellness. Through this holistic pathway, individuals not only improve their physical health, they also open the door to deeper spiritual growth and happiness. Through the wisdom of Buddhism, we discover that our bodies are not merely vessels, but temples deserving of reverence and kindness. The journey to physical wellness, then, becomes a path not just to living longer, but towards living a more fulfilling life.

Chapter 5. Mind-Body Synergy: The Spiritual Fitness Balance

Buddhist philosophy advocates that true wellness is a blend of harmony, spirituality, physical health, and mental clarity. To reach optimal health, a person must find balance in each of these fields. This unique approach to health and wellness, coined as the Mind-Body Synergy in this report, evolves beyond crunching abs and lifting weights. It fosters the intersection of three critical facets: physical exercise, mental strength, and spiritual notions.

5.1. Physical Exercise: The Pillar of Strength

Physical fitness is the foundation of wellness. It is the most tangible and perceptible aspect of health. When we think of fitness, it's traditionally associated with vigorous and strenuous exercise, like running, cycling, and lifting weights. But the imperative question lies here: Is pushing your body to its limits the only way to physical strength and health?

Buddhism offers a different perspective. It implores us to treat our bodies like temples and cherish them through nurturing acts rather than punishing ordeals. This chastening discipline promotes low-impact exercises such as walking, tai chi, and yoga. These gentle routines focus on fluid movements, boosting flexibility, stamina, and overall strength, and encouraging the body to move in sync with the mind's rhythm.

5.2. Mental Health: The Crucible of Wellness

Buddha highlighted the instrumental significance of a healthy mind: "To keep the body in good health is a duty...otherwise, we shall not be able to keep our mind strong and clear." Mental health carries an undeniable weight in defining a person's overall wellness.

Acknowledging the mind's health is about discovering balance within yourself, managing stress, honing focus, nurturing self-awareness, and cultivating positive emotions. Mindful meditation and meditative movements are key strategies to foster mental well-being. Instilling regular meditation and instrospection practices helps in identifying your thoughts, emotions, and beliefs, leading to increased self-awareness. As self-awareness improves, it aids in the growth of emotional intelligence, fostering a state of mental tranquility and resilience against mental or emotional disturbances.

5.3. Spiritual Fitness: The Beacon of Enlightenment

Spiritual fitness, while elusive and personal, provides sustenance to the roots of wellness. It is neither about being religious nor beholden to a higher power, but it refers to the pursuit of understanding your purpose in life and aligning your actions accordingly.

The practice of spiritual fitness in Buddhism constitutes meditation, mindfulness, and radiating compassion and kindness towards oneself and others. Spirituality encourages living in the present moment, as Buddha once said, "Do not dwell in the past, do not dream of the future, concentrate the mind on the present moment."

These practices ensure we live a life that is in unison with our values and lowers stress while promoting positive relationships. The ultimate goal is to attain inner peace—a deep calmness transcending physical health and mental health, leading to a feeling of satisfaction, meaning, and purpose in life.

5.4. Attaining the Spiritual Fitness Balance: A Practical Approach

Attaining the spiritual fitness balance entails weaving together the fabric of physical exercise, mental wellbeing, and spiritual enlightenment. Though each of these elements is essential on its own, their combined effect holds a profound impact on a person's overall health, planting the seeds for a sound mind in a sound body.

Daily Habits for Mind-Body Synergy

1. Practise a form of physical exercise that aligns with your body's rhythm, strengths, and weaknesses. Yoga, walking, tai chi, or other types of low-impact exercises are great choices.

2. Incorporate meditation into your daily schedule. Even a few minutes daily goes a long way in improving focus and mental clarity.

3. Engage in mindful activities – like mindful eating and mindful walking. It forms a path to connect with your inner self while keeping you rooted in the present moment.

4. Regular self-reflection is key. Journaling or introspection helps in understanding your thoughts, motivations, and actions.

5. Exercise compassion and kindness, not only toward others but importantly, toward yourself.

Inculcating these habits is the first step towards achieving mind-body synergy.

5.5. Not Just an Exercise, But a Way of Life

It is crucial to comprehend that the spiritual fitness balance is more than a workout routine. Treat it as a holistic approach to living healthfully, harmoniously, and wisely. Its aim extends beyond weight loss and muscle gain. It implores to cultivate respect, care, and love for your body, mind, and soul, and upholds wellness as a way of life–a journey to be relished rather than a finish line to be crossed.

As our understanding of health and wellbeing evolves, we learn that physical strength does not solely define fitness. True fitness comes from a mindful and holistic approach, integrating physical strength, mental clarity, and spiritual awareness into your lifestyle. So heed Buddha's wisdom and make your journey to fitness, one of compassion, mindfulness, and balance—personifying the ethos of our Special Report "Buddha's Guide to Fitness: The Path to Mindful and Holistic Health".

Chapter 6. Meditative Moves: Training into Tranquility

Before we can tread on the path to wellness, it's essential to delve into the philosophy that forms its bedrock. Synthesizing the wisdom of Buddha's teachings with the science of physical fitness, a unique blend of meditative movement arises, providing a path into tranquility. What follows is a detailed exploration into the depths of this philosophy, presenting actionable practices and marking checkpoints for your personal journey.

6.1. Understanding Meditative Moves

Meditative Moves refers to an amalgamation of mind and body exercises that trickle tranquility in your being. Unifying the principles of Buddha's mindfulness teachings with modern movement science, we stretch beyond purely physical benefits to embrace mental and spiritual growth.

While normal exercise focuses on physical strength and endurance, Meditative Moves goes an extra mile. It encourages you to become more present, feeling and respect each movement, noticing how your body reacts and adapts. The union of physical exercise and mental mindfulness grants a peaceful rhythm to your practice, helping you cultivate inner silence and tranquility within the clamor of daily life.

6.2. The Intersection of Mindfulness and Movement

Building upon Buddha's teachings of mindfulness, Meditative Moves introduce a new dimension to exercise. Mindfulness is all about being present in the moment, aware of our body, emotions, and thoughts. Introducing this into our fitness regime, we encourage complete engagement in each movement.

This intersection of mindfulness with movement amplifies the benefits of exercise, going beyond simple strength and flexibility to include stress reduction, improved focus, and suppressed anxiety – all pivotal in battling the perils of modern living. By channeling your core energy into each workout session, mindfulness paves the path for a holistically healthy lifestyle.

6.3. Incorporating Meditative Moves into Your Routine

Those new to the concept of Meditative Moves might feel daunted. However, with consistent practice, mastering the art of mindful movements can be enlightening. Here's a step-by-step guide to incorporating meditative moves into your daily routine:

1. Start by choosing a quiet and comfortable spot where you will not be easily distracted. This space will serve as your sanctuary while practicing Meditative Moves.

2. Begin each session by spending a few minutes in silence, focusing on your breath. This phase is vital in preparing your mind for a more centered workout.

3. Once your mind is calm, start your exercise. Be mindful of every movement, dedicating your full attention to the process. Feel the energy flow through your muscles and pay close attention to your body's responses.

4. Always remember, the goal of Meditative Moves is not to reach the highest intensity or the toughest phase but to feel a deeper connection with your own body.

5. End your exercise with a few more minutes of silence, reflecting

on your workout and noticing any changes in your mind and
body.

6.4. Exercises Under the Umbrella of Meditative Moves

Meditative Moves is not restricted to a specific set of exercises. A
myriad of workouts can be adapted to incorporate mindfulness,
inducing a peaceful rhythm to your regime. Among them, Tai Chi,
Yoga, Qigong, Pilates and even simple forms of aerobic exercises such
as walking or swimming can be performed mindfully.

Each form of exercise mentioned grants specific benefits. While yoga
and Pilates deliver excellent strength and flexibility training, Tai Chi
and Qigong are lauded for stress reduction and boosting mental
health. Aerobic exercises, performed mindfully, not only improve
cardiovascular health but also infuse a sense of peace and calm.

6.5. Measuring Progress

The beauty of Meditative Moves is that the definition of progress
extends beyond mere physical metrics. Besides observing
improvements in strength, flexibility or stamina, keep track of
changes in your stress levels, self-awareness and general feelings of
tranquility.

It's this subtle yet profound elevation into a state of calm and
serenity that indicates progress. You grow – not only as someone
physically fit but also attain a tranquil state of mind that Buddha
himself advocated for.

6.6. Conclusion: The Path to Lasting Tranquility

Meditative Moves are more than a unique blend of physical movements with mindfulness. They represent a lifestyle, a bridge that connects the physicality of our existence with the realms of our mind and spirit. Infusing Buddha's teachings into our modern fitness routines, we birth a harmonious blend of mindfulness and motion, furnishing a path to lasting tranquility.

Remember, the goal here isn't just an improved physique, but holistic wellness, a harmonious and uplifting symphony of mind, body, and spirit. Practice Meditative Moves consistently, explore its depths, and you'll uncover a wellspring of tranquility within yourself - steady, overwhelming, and beautiful in its depth. The path may be intricate, but the reward – a tranquil mind in a strong body – is worth every step.

Chapter 7. The Middle Path: Avoiding Extremes in Fitness

The Middle Way is a concept in Buddhism that signifies a path of moderation away from the extremes of self-indulgence and self-mortification. Similarly, in the realm of fitness, the key to long-term wellness corresponds to walking the middle path—a balance between overexertion and idleness. The practical implications of the Middle Way in fitness revolve around integrating a moderate, regular, and varied physical fitness routine that effectively unites the body, the mind, and the spirit into a harmonious whole.

7.1. The Illusion of Extremes in Fitness

One of the key challenges in today's fitness scene is the dichotomous framing of exercise. Arbitrary goals are often set, making fitness seem like a challenge to be conquered—a mountain to climb, or a foe to defeat. These metaphors embody extreme attitudes towards both ends of the spectrum, the excessive and the insufficient.

Extreme physical training, often construed as the epitome of fitness, can potentially cause physical stress and injuries. Simultaneously, on the other side, avoiding physical activity, often associated with comfort and leisure, can lead to obesity and associated medical conditions.

Thus, the Middle Path in fitness is absolutely critical—it teaches us that neither extreme is efficient or sustainable. The path of moderation lies in maintaining a balanced lifestyle, intertwining sufficient exercise, healthy nutritional habits, recovery, and mental well-being.

7.2. The Middle Way Mentality in Practical Fitness

The task is not to eradicate the extremes, but to acknowledge their existence as elements of a larger fitness scale. The Middle Path helps to recalibrate and balance their predominance in one's life.

To act upon this, we should take into consideration exercise frequency, intensity, time, and type—commonly referred to as the F.I.T.T Principle. Keeping routines flexible when it comes to these aspects will not only prevent the action from becoming a dreaded chore but will also ensure that fitness can easily be a regular and enjoyable part of our everyday life.

1. Frequency: The aim should be to engage in moderate exercises most days of the week, keeping in mind to listen to the body and allowing it to rest when required. Rest aids muscle recovery, and maintaining a balance between activity and recovery forms the crux of the Middle Way in fitness.

2. Intensity: It is crucial to vary the intensity of workouts—incorporating high-intensity and low-intensity routines into your regimen. This variety in intensity ensures that the body does not adapt to a particular type of stress, which can often lead to a fitness plateau.

3. Time: Time spent on fitness should not be a point of stress. Quality should always be prioritized over quantity. Even if time spent on a specific exercise session is brief, it can still contribute positively to overall health, demonstrating that moderate time dedicated to regular fitness can yield substantial benefits.

4. Type: Engaging in a variety of exercise types is critical for overall body conditioning. From yoga to weightlifting, every exercise has its unique benefits. It's also necessary to ensure that fitness routine includes elements of strength training, cardio, flexibility, and balance training.

This intrinsic balance found in the Middle Way encourages us to avoid seeing exercise as a punishing experience or as an escape from reality. Instead, it transforms fitness into a practice that enhances quality of life, keeping us engaged, and positively motivated.

7.3. Conscious Eating and The Middle Path

The Middle Way, in terms of diet, rejects harsh dietary restrictions and overindulgence. It embraces mindful eating—a practice focused on enjoying food and understanding the signals that our body sends us about hunger and fullness. The Middle Way in diet aids in creating a healthy relationship with food, one where guilt and shame don't play a role.

Balancing nutrition is vital—ensuring a mix of macro and micronutrients, including all essential food groups in our meals, and adjusting the quantities based on our lifestyle requirements. Avoiding extreme diets which delete entire food groups promotes a more sustainable approach towards dietary habits. Spaces for occasional indulgences, what is often termed as 'cheat days', may also help in maintaining a healthy balance.

The road to optimum health cannot exclude diet or fitness; the Middle Path helps us understand the interconnectedness of these elements and the significance of maintaining equilibrium between them.

7.4. The Middle Path and Mental Health

Physical fitness does not exist in a vacuum; it coexists dynamically with mental health. The Middle Path underscores the significance of taking care of our minds alongside our bodies. It includes incorporating mindful practices— meditation, breathing exercises, yoga—which help cultivate a sense of inner peace, vital for our overall well-being.

The benefit of exercise on mental health is widely known. Regular physical activity can reduce anxiety, combat depression, and boost mood. Thus, consistency in moderate exercise can have a profound impact on mental well-being, illuminating the fact that the path to good health isn't a straight, narrow path, but one that meanders through the physical, mental, and spiritual terrains of human existence.

7.5. Conclusion

The Middle Path in fitness isn't about perfection but about balance. It involves understanding our bodies, recognizing our limits, and pushing ourselves within these limits. It celebrates progress over perfection, persistence over instant gratification, and mindfulness over mindless exertion.

Above all, the Middle Path reiterates the need for us to embrace fitness as part of our life, as a practice that nourishes not just our bodies, but also our minds and spirits. The Middle Path represents a comprehensive, inclusive, and holistic approach to fitness and wellness.

Chapter 8. Outer Strength, Inner Peace: Enriching Workouts with Mindfulness

Holistic health requires harmonizing every dimension of human wellness, including the mental and the physical. A vital way to attain this harmony is through mindful exercise, embedding the wisdom of Buddhism into your fitness routine. This practice can strengthen your body while fostering mental serenity, embodying the ancient adage that a healthy body houses a healthy mind.

8.1. The Symbiosis of Mind and Body

Every step you take, every breath in, every rep out — every physical action is intertwined with your mind. Our body and mind are not two distinct entities. Rather, they form a interconnected ecosystem, each influencing the other. The rising discipline of psychoneuroimmunology underscores this connection, underscoring how our thoughts and feelings can impact our physical health. Conversely, physical activity releases endorphins, the brain's feel-good neurotransmitters, thereby fostering a sense of wellbeing.

Mindful exercise leverages this symbiosis, uniting physical activity with conscious attention to one's body, thoughts, and emotions. The tenets of mindfulness and Buddhism enhance your workouts by turning them into an opportunity for spiritual growth.

8.2. The Pillars of Mindful Exercise

There are several core principles that centralize mediation into exercise, for eventual benefits to physical, emotional, and mental health.

Presence: Maintaining awareness of the present moment is the backbone of mindful exercise. While it might be tempting to let your mind stray during a workout, try focusing on your breathing, the rhythm of your feet on the pavement, the sensation of your muscles contracting

Non-Judgment: Mindful exercise is not about setting personal records or comparing oneself to others. It is about appreciating your body for what it is and what it can do at that moment. Do not berate yourself for a slow run or a missed lift; instead, acknowledge the effort it took to simply show up and maintain the commitment to your health.

Patience: Mindfulness is a skill, and it takes time to develop. You might not experience noticeable changes right away, but stay patient. Just like physical strength, inner peace is accrued incrementally.

8.3. Incorporating Mindfulness into Your Workout Routine

Creating a mindful workout routine doesn't require monumental shifts. A few minor adjustments and a change in your mindset can greatly augment your exercise experience.

Pre-workout meditation: Begin by meditating for a couple of minutes before your workout. Sit in a comfortable position, close your eyes, and focus on deep, steady breathing. This helps center your mind and prepares your body for movement.

Focusing on the body: During the workout, stay connected with your body. Pay attention to your form, the engagement of your muscles, and your body's response to the exertion. This practice not only improves the effectiveness of the workout by ensuring correct technique, but also enhances self-awareness.

Post-workout reflection: After your workout, take a few moments to meditate and reflect on the exercise session. How did the workout make you feel physically and emotionally? Did you learn anything about your body or mind? This time for reflection can deepen your relationship with exercising and motivate further progress.

8.4. Reframing Exercise as a Path to Enlightenment

When we connect our fitness journey with our spiritual goal, our mindset shifts. Exercise is no longer a chore or a selfish indulgence, but an integral part of our quest for enlightenment and self-improvement. Every moment on the mat or in the gym, instead of being a struggle, becomes a revelation, a chance to discover yourself, to push your boundaries, and to cultivate inner peace.

By incorporating the teachings of Buddha into your fitness journey, you're not only sculpting a healthier body, but also cultivating a fiercely resilient, positive mind. You will learn to approach your workouts with gratitude, recognizing them as a unique opportunity to improve both your physical and mental prowess. A sense of balance, serenity, and empowering self-awareness are just a touch away — ingrained within each step, each rep, each breath.

Overall, a fitness journey enriched with mindfulness and the wisdom of Buddhism is not merely a path to a healthier body, but a journey towards the grandeur of self-understanding and peace. As we cultivate our external strength, our internal peace blossoms, fostering a life of balance, health, and holistic wellness.

Chapter 9. Holistic Healing: A Buddha Inspired Wellness Journey

In this undertaking of holistic healing, we embark on a riveting journey envisaged by Buddha, an inspiration that draws upon mindfulness, meditation, and balance, all playing central roles in wellness. It takes the integrated approach to health, where the mind, body, and spirit are not just interconnected but essentially one.

9.1. Understanding the Buddha's Philosophy

The Buddha presented the Eightfold Path to guide individuals towards enlightenment, sharing insights about right mindfulness, right action, and right view, amongst others. This shows an inherent focus on the overall wellbeing and balance in life attributes that are central to comprehensive health.

Our health is often determined by our actions, thoughts, and perspectives, and it only makes sense to harness these elements to achieve holistic health. Buddha's teachings remind us to be present and conscious in every action, be it having a meal, going for a run, or simply breathing. Mindfulness brings an overwhelming array of benefits, from stress reduction to improved focus, all contributing to better health.

In addition, Buddha's school of thought significantly emphasized on compassion, including self-compassion. Much of our health journey involves being kind to ourselves, loving our bodies, respecting our limitations, and celebrating our victories, however small.

9.2. Integrating Mindful Movement

Mindful movement – the practice of consciously focusing on your body as it moves – takes center stage in the Buddha's approach to physical wellness. This technique transcends the boundaries of traditional exercise, allowing practitioners to achieve physical fitness while also fostering mental and spiritual growth.

Physical activities like yoga, tai chi, or mindful walking, which requires you to tune into each movement and remain aware of your body, offer both an exercise for your body and a form of meditation. These movements, when performed diligently and regularly, can lead to improved flexibility, strength, and body awareness. At the same time, they cultivate mindfulness, enhance the connection between mind and body, and open the door to a greater understanding of one's self.

9.3. The Role of Nutrition

Buddha's teachings encourage a mindful approach towards what we eat. Following the Middle Way, Buddha suggests eating what is necessary without falling sway to either self-indulgence or self-denial. This mindfulness does not simply refer to choosing healthy, nutritious food, but also appreciating the taste, understanding the origins and being grateful for the sustenance it provides.

One of the principles of the Buddhist philosophy about food is moderation. Overeating can lead to physical discomfort and metabolic imbalance, while starving oneself deprives the body of its necessary nutrients. Therefore, a balance is essential in maintaining good health and vitality.

9.4. The Power of Meditation and Mindfulness

Meditation, one of the pillars of Buddha's teachings, yields a wealth of benefits for mental and physical health. Regular meditation can help reduce anxiety, control stress, improve focus, and facilitate a better understanding of your own mind.

Meditation enables you to develop greater mindfulness – a state of being fully present and engaged in the current moment. Not only does mindfulness promote mental wellbeing, but it also enhances your physical health by boosting immune response and decreasing inflammation.

Mindfulness translates to fitness too. By being mindful during workouts, you can focus on your form, aligning your movements perfectly, making each moment count, improving performance, and reducing the risk of injury.

9.5. Healing Emotionally

Buddha's teachings weren't just carved for their philosophical value but their innate therapeutic potential as well. Emotional wellness is a major component of holistic health, and Buddha's wisdom can undeniably guide us there.

The Buddha urges us to accept and acknowledge emotions, not suppress them, facilitating emotional wellbeing. Practicing mindfulness helps keep a close check on our emotional health by reminding us to live in the moment. It aids in managing and processing our feelings constructively, not letting them accumulate and impact our mental peace.

9.6. Compassion and Connectivity

The Buddha's teachings often highlight interconnectedness, reminding us of how connected our minds, bodies, and spirits are, and how our actions can affect others and the world around us. This sense of connectivity fosters compassion, not just towards others, but towards ourselves.

Compassion in our physical fitness journey allows us to listen to our body, to give it the care it needs, and to provide it with challenges that facilitate growth, without crossing the boundaries of self-love.

In conclusion, Buddha's wisdom grant us a guide to navigating the path to holistic health. These practices of mindfulness, compassion, and balance work collectively to promote better physical health, mental clarity, emotional stability, and a deep connection with the self and the world around us. As you experience a wellness journey inspired by Buddha, remember, it's not just about the destination. Each step, each moment is a vital part of the journey itself. So are the insights, realizations, and transformations you undergo along the way. These embody the true essence of Buddha's enlightened path to holistic health.

Chapter 10. Reflective Recuperation: Mindful Recovery and Self-Care

The pursuit of physical wellness need not be shrouded with rigorous strain and prolonged exhaustion. In fact, the journey towards holistic health values the process of recovery as foundational as the efforts exerted in workout regimes. This underpins the necessity for reflective recuperation, the act of consciously immersing oneself in mindful recovery and self-care.

10.1. The Imperative of Recovery

Rest forms the linchpin of sustainable physical fitness. The body replenishes itself during periods of quietude following strenuous activities. This relaxation allows the body to rebuild tissues, reduces stress levels, and enhances overall physical performance. Bear in mind that effective downtime doesn't suggest launching into complete dormancy, but actively embracing activities that foster repair and rejuvenation. The integration of mindfulness into this process amplifies the benefits, reinforcing the interconnection between the body and the mind.

10.2. Embracing Mindfulness in Recovery

Mindfulness is the practice of focusing one's awareness on the present moment, calmly acknowledging and accepting one's feelings, thoughts, and bodily sensations. When integrated into your recovery routine, mindfulness can assist in the attunement to bodily signals, fostering a deeper understanding of your physical needs, and promoting a more efficient healing process.

10.3. Practicing Mindful Breathing

One of the most effective ways to incorporate mindfulness into recovery is through mindful breathing, a technique that merely necessitates your focus on the inhalation and exhalation process. This practice encourages relaxation and healing by triggering the body's natural relaxation response, helping to reduce muscle tension and psychological stress.

10.4. Mindful Yoga for Recovery

While restorative yoga forms the centuries-old discipline's restful side, it's an exceptionally potent tool for recovery, promoting both physical recuperation and mental relaxation. The practice emphasizes prolonged poses that encourage your muscles to relax, mitigating strain and enhancing flexibility. Mindfully engaging in these positions, concentrating keenly on your breath, and observing your thoughts can profoundly influence your recovery process.

10.5. The Art of Mindful Eating

In the context of recovery, mindful eating plays a critical role. By giving careful consideration to the nutrients you consume post-exercise, and mindfully enjoying every bite, the body and mind can undergo a more effective regeneration process.

10.6. The Role of Sleep in Recovery

Quality sleep is vital for a holistic healing process. Mindful preparation for sleep, including the practice of calming activities like light reading, meditation, or a gentle walk, can greatly impact sleep quality and hence, recovery.

10.7. Self-Care as a Form of Recovery

Valuing self-care is instrumental in reflective recuperation. The embrace of skincare routines, soothing baths, or listening to calming music, all play definitive roles in facilitating a mindful recovery process.

Rest, they say, is as significant as action. Similarly, the phase of recovery is as essential in your fitness journey as your workout routine. By adopting a mindful approach towards relaxing, you form a graceful synergy between physical exertiveness and profound restfulness, reinforcing your path to a healthy and enlightened existence. While pushing your body past its limits can yield strength and stamina, a genuinely enlightened fitness journey acknowledges the harmony of exertion and restfulness, making reflective recuperation an integral element in achieving holistic health.

Chapter 11. Cultivating Spiritual Endurance: The Buddha's Approach to Resilience

Resting in the lap of tranquility, Buddhism offers a rich tapestry of concepts and principles that can contribute substantially to our understanding of resilience. Delving into Buddha's teachings, one can glean that resilience is more than mere earthly grit or fortitude; it is a journey inward, a constant flow of energy and wisdom, rippling outwards to impact all facets of reality.

11.1. The Tenets of Buddhism and Resilience

Buddha's teachings can be distilled into a few key principles: The Four Noble Truths and The Eightfold Path. Each of these enhances our understanding and response to suffering, fortifying our internal strength and resilience.

The Four Noble Truths encompass the essence of Buddha's teachings. They are: the truth of suffering (Dukkha), the truth of the cause of suffering (Samudaya), the truth of the end of suffering (Nirodha), and the truth of the path to the end of suffering (Magga). These truths guide us to acknowledge our struggles, understand their origin, ascertain the possibility of overcoming them, and finally set us on the path to do so.

The Eightfold Path, meanwhile, elucidates the practical steps to liberate ourselves from suffering and fortify our inner resilience. Each step – right understanding, right thought, right speech, right action, right livelihood, right effort, right mindfulness, and right concentration – forms an essential component of this path.

11.2. A Deeper Understanding of Resilience

In the Buddha's teachings, resilience isn't merely about overcoming obstacles; it's about understanding and accepting their existence, their transient nature, and thereby not being perturbed by their presence.

The process of cultivating spiritual endurance necessitates grasping the impermanent nature of things. Known as Anicca in Buddhism, this concept allows us to comprehend that change is part of life. By internalizing these teachings, we learn to healthily cope with situations that are beyond our control, foster equanimity in the face of adversity, and base our happiness on inner peace rather than external circumstances.

11.3. Resilience in Practice

The mark of true resilience is to encounter suffering, understand it, and endure it with grace. To achieve this, one must first accept that adversity is a part of life. This acceptance, inspired by the First Noble Truth, catalyzes the transformation of our mind, making us more resilient to life's tribulations.

Next, we trace the roots of our struggles and eliminate them. The Second Noble Truth, Samudaya, prompts us to understand how our own desires and aversions contribute to our suffering. This investigative approach allows us to understand our role in our struggle and encourages a proactive approach towards mental wellness.

Engaging the Third Noble Truth, Nirodha, enlightenment is

understood as the ultimate cessation of suffering. The mind immersed in Dhamma can experience peace amidst chaos, attaining an unshakable mental fortitude that withstands life's challenges.

Lastly, employing the Fourth Noble Truth, Magga, sets us on the Eightfold Path. Together, these Eight Steps form a pragmatic framework for developing resilience through ethical principles, meditation, and wisdom.

11.4. Cultivating Resilience through Meditation

An indispensable tool in fostering resilience is meditation. It incorporates the facets of mindfulness and concentration: both instruments used to hone our internal vigilance, reduce pressure, and enhance focus. With practice, meditation gives us insight into the real nature of life and bolsters our ability to graciously navigate life's ebbs and flows.

In viewing resilience through the Buddha's lens, we not just encounter a dynamic system for dealing with adversary but also an enlightened path brimming with wisdom and inner peace. Internalizing these teachings enables us to experience profound transformation, bolstering our resilience – a spiritual endurance that allows us to navigate life's turbulences with grace, equanimity, and an unruffled mind.